A BUSINESS OF HEALING

A BUSINESS OF HEALING

THE DIRECT EXPERIENCE OF AN ENERGETIC
PRACTITIONER

JERI LAWSON

INTENTION PRESS

ISBN: 978-1-7355453-0-1 (print)

ISBN: 978-1-7355453-1-8 (e-book)

Dedicated to Terese Allara and Neal Lowen.
Thank you for giving me the space to hold space for others.

CONTENTS

"There is no distinction between the one who gives, the one who receives, and the gift itself."
–Thich Nhat Hanh

INTRODUCTION

THIS BOOK IS ABOUT MY EXPERIENCE AS A PROFESSIONAL healer over the last twenty-five years.

This is not a book about the euphoria of healing. There are plenty of wonderful and inspiring books written on Reiki, Healing Touch, and other energetic modalities. This book is about issues and paradoxes in my practice that I couldn't find in books by other healers, things that took me a long time to understand on my own.

It is about how I learned to trust the healing process and let go of everything blocking me from being fully present for my clients. How I learned to hold an energetic space that would allow others to self-heal. How my obsessive spiritual seeking ended.

This book is about how I learned to navigate the practical daily aspects of being self-employed while holding a sacred space for people who are healing from cancer. It's about spiritual expectations, the evolving practice of self-care, and how I learned to stay grounded while holding a space for the vast possibilities of untapped human potential. This is the book I would have wanted to read when I was starting my practice.

You would think that when a client who is "dying" from cancer suddenly goes into full remission, it would be easy to accept the healing as a wonderful thing. Yet, when another client didn't "heal" in the same way, I couldn't help but feel like I had somehow failed. As I opened up to how powerful this work is, the more responsibility for my clients' healing I seemed to take on.

Sometimes even simple things became overwhelming for periods of time. Once I was shopping at Walgreens after a morning of two beautiful, heart-opening Reiki sessions and discovered the fluorescent lights suddenly made me sick, like bolt-out-the-door sick.

Having a healing business is about connecting with another human being in the most profound, intimate moments of life in unity consciousness, and then afterward asking for something as mundane and materialistic as money. This book is how I learned to hold space for all of it.

My intention is not to tell you how to heal, or what you should experience in a session, but to give you the confidence to let the energy guide you in opening to your unique abilities as you start your healing practice. What you think should happen, and what actually happens in a healing, could be very different things. The direct experience of your healing sessions is where you can discover the portal to that healing place where all possibilities exist. The possibilities for you and your client.

This book was initially inspired by conversations with healer and client Heather Swallow. Heather had been struggling with severe depression for most of her life. She was on five medications for anxiety and depression when she came to me for her first healing. She had also been given a myriad of misleading diagnoses.

Using my pendulum at that first session to check her energy centers, I found all her chakras were open except the crown chakra at the top of her head—her connection to spirit. I remember thinking to myself, "Could this be it?"

It might have been. Once she was connected to her higher self, her intuition opened and with regular healing sessions her life turned around pretty fast.

One year after her initial visit, she started her own thriving healing practice and accomplished in two years what had taken me twenty. She has found her work in the world and financially supports her family with her healing practice. Her clients are thriving and she is holding the same space for others that I hold for her. It is a joy to witness.

Heather decided I was her mentor. One thing led to another and now I am "mentoring" a few other clients as they discover their healing abilities and sustain their healing practices. These are the stories and the discoveries in my practice that appeared to have helped Heather and other healers.

The world needs more healers. More energetic practitioners available to go to hospitals, nursing homes, hospice centers, and shelters. I have witnessed how energetic healing sessions can bring so much comfort to so many people. I hope this book inspires others to take a class and explore their healing gifts.

I found that human beings are much more powerful

than we realize. We have only just scratched the surface of the vast possibilities of human potential. Opening to our energetic abilities is one way of discovering how to heal ourselves and heal others emotionally, mentally, and physically. Connecting to our deepest intuition and our highest wisdom is available right here and right now.

DISCLAIMER

EVERYTHING IS CHANGING AND EVOLVING IN EVERY MOMENT. The only constant is the direct experience of this present moment. All opinions, information, advice, insights, working models, and even how I tell these stories may change at any time.

As my perspective shifts, everything shifts. Acknowledging and living from this constantly evolving energy is the foundation of this book. This book is like a snapshot of time, a moment in my evolving practice.

1

THE QUESTION

A CLIENT ONCE ASKED ME, "WHAT DO YOU EXPERIENCE during a healing session?"

That short question inspired a very long answer. An answer which is very fluid and is constantly evolving with every session.

Before I begin, it might be helpful to first describe what I do as a healer and how the energy is showing up for my clients.

My job as a healer is to hold the energetic space my client needs to self-heal. All healing is self-healing.

In my sessions at this time, I find myself doing long, slow Chakra Connections as taught in the Healing Touch Program. A Chakra Connection is a full-body technique that starts at the feet and ends above the head. It facilitates connecting, opening, and balancing all energy systems with a series of hand placements over the major energy centers of the body. I usually start at the feet and end at the top of the head.

I am primarily kinesthetic in my perception of energy. I feel color, energy moving, and blocks in the human aura with my hands. Sometimes I also see light, as well as feel and hear vibrations, tones, and other sounds. At times I may feel things in my own body that give me information about what is happening in my client's body—like my throat will feel scratchy for about thirty seconds, or I will be aware of my ankle throbbing for a minute.

Every session is different; no two sessions have ever been alike. Clients I see every week have a different experience each time. I still find this remarkable, even after twenty-five years of having a healing practice.

When I first started healing work, I often perceived energies moving through me and through the room. Like a stream of grounding honey/yellow energy for one client, or a wave of cooling, clear blue for another. Every so often I still perceive energy like that, but for the last eight years there has usually been a specific frequency or space that fills the whole room for each client. In this space, everything that my client needs in that moment unfolds for them. This healing space can be deeply still, yet, is never stagnant. It morphs and evolves throughout the session.

I am generally mentally clear and noting what I am experiencing during the treatment, as well as tracking how my client is doing. Yet, there are healing states that are so encompassing that I can't find where "I" end and "they" begin.

There are times when it feels like the whole room is underwater and my arms can only move slowly and heavily from one hand position to another. In this state, the energy feels like waves flowing through both me and the client in this weighted, fluid space. It's like we are deep under the ocean where everything is water, and everything is connected. Even my thoughts are slow, and it feels like they take a long time to form and then dissolve.

Some sessions are so ethereal that I feel like I am healing a cloud, not another human body. I can feel the bright translucent light and once in a while see it in the room. I do not have, or have not yet opened up to the ability to communicate directly with guides and angels, yet I almost always sense other distinct healing presences in the room. These presences have always been extremely helpful. Many of my clients tell me after the healing who or what they saw, or how many sets of hands they felt.

Some healings create a very sparkly light in the room. In others, I am kinesthetically aware of a very low tone or vibration permeating everything. Occasionally I may suddenly feel intensely sleepy. That is an energetic frequency that may last most of the session, or only a few minutes. When that happens, I have to focus on my breath, sit even more upright, and stay balanced until it passes. The sleepy energy has proven to be greatly beneficial for my clients, especially when I stopped resisting it.

Sometimes the healing is mostly about balancing my client's physical body, and I am experiencing the healing energy with my hands. I might sense the energy gently unwinding in circular patterns under my palms at each hand position. Sometimes I am very aware of my client's cranial pulse, and that is the prominent guiding sensation for me during the session.

Once in a while the energy feels electric—like a pulse between my palms. Sometimes there is a magnetic pull throughout the session in one direction, as if through the session I am pushing my client to the right or left. Often there is a sense of expansion—like the area between my hands is filling up as if bread is rising. I have felt my hands merge with the client's body, like there are no hands and no body, just this space where my hands should be.

I have become aware of my client's energy field as a collection of frequencies that are subtly harmonizing. Like all the individual musicians in an orchestra tuning up before a concert. Every time I change my hand position, I sense a different tone. It's like I am feeling sound. My clients are tuning themselves in the sacred space.

Almost all sessions move through several different energetic states in the same treatment.

Time is usually not linear in a healing. I have to periodically check the clock, which is right by the healing table, so I know how much time I have left in the session. My subjective experience of time is not reliable at all. I can't tell you how many times I have looked at the clock after what feels like only ten minutes and find thirty minutes have gone by.

Time can also "jump." I will just realize one moment that I wasn't there. That maybe both the client and I skipped out for a split second or a few minutes. I can't be sure, since I was not there to experience it. I am still uncomfortable with suddenly not being in my healing session, even if only for a moment, but after a few years of this occurring I decided to just go with it. It appears when this kind of energy shift happens it is very, very healing for my client.

A few times, I have sensed my client entraining with my energy field—the synchronization of their body rhythm to mine. This has only happened a handful of times and it is more of a physical connection, rather than an energetic one.

I would say energy is like water. During a session it may be hard, like ice, or misty like a fog. Sometimes it's heavy like a milkshake, and other times it's clear and clean like water from a spring. The energy of the session can be totally encompassing, like when the healing space suddenly feels like I am at the bottom of the ocean. Sometimes it's moving like a large river, or even a water-fall. Then sometimes it can feel totally still.

I could go on and on, but I think this gives you an idea of what I may be experiencing when holding a healing space for my client. Everything I have described always feels perfect during the treatment and makes so much sense in the moment—like I knew it all beforehand, or I am just remembering it as it arises. I almost always feel peaceful and *grateful* after each session.

2

STILLNESS IS PROFOUND

IT IS *VERY* IMPORTANT TO REMIND PRACTITIONERS AND clients that if you don't have any of the experiences I have just written about, it is not because you are not an effective healer, or you are not receiving the most profound session possible for you at this moment.

> *My experience during a healing session may have nothing to do with how beneficial the treatment is for my client.*

This sounds illogical, but it is true for me. It took me years to understand this.

Many of the most life-changing, profound sessions for my clients have also been the ones that are experienced as completely still.

> *"I felt SO much better after our session yesterday. It almost surprised me how much better I felt, because nothing huge or dramatic happened during the session.*

Remarkably, by the time I left yesterday, I felt completely rested despite getting only half a night's sleep. Some of the irritability and stress had lifted too. Thank you!"

— CLIENT AFTER A SESSION

"There were so many different things going on in our session. I swear—every time you shifted to a different part of my body, my experience changed entirely. The one thing that was consistent was that there was a quietness (I wanted initially to say stillness, but that was not the right word) that moved through me. It wasn't any kind of movement or vibration or heat or anything; it felt most closely like those really still rivers—the way the water can be almost flat but still moving. That's sort of what it felt like running through me the entire time. There were moments of heat and warmth, but not really much more intense energy than quiet movement."

— CLIENT AFTER A SESSION

There are several healing modalities, teachers, and lineages of Reiki that suggest you not become distracted by sensations, thoughts or imagination, no matter how phenomenal or engaging during the healing. The practice is to stay calm, centered, grounded and focused.

One of the greatest teachers I have studied with, Frans Stiene, writes about this. I still wish I could say that all my sessions are deeply still, yet my personal experience is that sensations, movement, and thoughts still arise in the healing space. Maybe that will change, maybe that is just how my unique abilities work best. What I am sure of is that the most powerful thing I can do for my client is simply not resist, judge, block or attach to anything that happens in the healing space.

> *"By being still everything is illuminated. When every-thing is illuminated there is no difference anymore between stillness and movement."*

> — FRANS STIENE, COPYRIGHT
> INTERNATIONAL: HOUSE OF REIKI
> WWW.IHREIKI.COM

3

LEARNING TO TRUST THE ENERGY

MY EXPERIENCE OF THE HEALING SPACE NOW IS VERY different from when I first started my healing practice. When I began my healing practice, at the beginning of each session I was usually too nervous to even feel my client's energy. In the Healing Touch Program we learn to document our treatments by diagnosing our client's biofield and chakras before and after the session. So I would start with a short Chakra Connection, or other full-body technique, and then I found I could feel and diagnose what was energetically going on in my client's aura.

My Healing Touch Mentor and Instructor, Carol Kinney, always said in her classes that she couldn't feel her client's energy in her first two years of practicing Healing Touch. She kept doing energy work because her client's responses to her sessions were so positive. I always found that reassuring.

For me, opening up to my own gifts and learning to trust the energy turned out to be a continual, never ending process of letting go of whatever was blocking me from the direct experience of my healing sessions.

This included letting go of performance anxiety when working with a new client and fear that my client will not benefit from the healing. Over the years I have learned to not attach to any thoughts or unconscious beliefs that I am not enough in any way. I have even let go of my expectations of how my clients should be benefiting from the sessions and, surprisingly, even my egoic desire to help my clients and relieve their suffering. That last discovery was quite unexpected.

> *It took me over twenty years to develop the ability to completely trust the energy. To understand that whatever happens during a healing is, and will always be, perfect. This trust has become an embodied skill. Now fully embedded in my muscle memory, this healing skill is my superpower.*

We are all capable of accessing our unique superpower, and it certainly does not need to take twenty years.

4

LETTING GO OF MY AGENDA

MY EGO LOVES AGENDAS. AS LONG AS I HAVE AN EGO, I WILL have agendas. I feel more comfortable and professional being prepared and having a sequence of techniques outlined in my mind before each session. A client I worked with many years ago taught me that trusting the energy often means dropping all my well-made plans as soon as the healing begins.

Jane was referred to me through her hospice nurse. She had stage four stomach cancer and was told that I could help her with the edema in her legs. Jane wanted to be able to keep walking up and down the stairs in her condo until the very end of her life.

The Lymphatic Drain is a powerful Healing Touch technique in which I can assist the client in clearing their lymphatic system and reduce swelling. It is one of the most complex sequences of hand positions I learned in the program, and I had previously used it only a few times after my initial training. I reviewed it the day before

I was to see Jane, excited to be able to help her walk in her last days at home.

I arrived at Jane's condo and carried my table upstairs. Jane was an atheist, originally from Brooklyn, New York, was passionate about art and had all her ducks in a row. She was upbeat, very alive and busy organizing piles of papers all over her bed. She told me exactly where she wanted me to put my massage table, pointed out a chair I could use if I needed it and explained exactly how the visit would progress. I liked her immediately.

Her husband, whom she had obviously loved dearly, had died about nine months earlier. Now that she was in hospice, she was getting her finances in order to leave her money to the art charities that meant so much to her. Jane was very excited about her donations. Once I had the massage table set up, she left her bed and paperwork and got on my table.

I had set my intention to help Jane physically with the swelling in her legs. As soon as I put my hands on her leg, I swear to God if felt like all hell broke loose in the room. It was the craziest thing I had ever witnessed up to that point during a healing. I felt like I was on a roller coaster—the room was a rocking and a rolling. The whirling and spinning lasted the whole session. It was all I could do to stay upright and hold the space. The Lymphatic Drain did not happen.

When the session was finished and the party was over, Jane was still in a trance state. I stood back and waited for her to open her eyes. I had no idea what I was going to say to her.

Lucky for me she did all the talking. She told me how her husband had come to visit during the healing; she was so happy and excited to connect with him again. I can't remember now how this impacted her view on life after death, but it was apparent she was very pleased with the session.

I still felt strangely guilty about not focusing on the edema and not doing the Lymphatic Drain technique. I did not feel like a well-trained and responsible healer. I went over the healing in my head for a long time afterward, and finally concluded there was nothing else I could have done. I had not been in charge of this session; I was just along for the ride. I was not comfortable with being in the backseat.

I saw Jane two weeks later. In between my visits she had a massage therapist give her a massage. After both the massage and the healing, she told me she could walk up and down her stairs by herself for the next three or four days, just as she wanted. There was obviously no need for me to feel guilty.

I didn't give Jane a Lymphatic Drain during the next treatment either, but that didn't seem to matter. The room broke out in energetic fireworks again as soon as I touched her body for a Chakra Connection. She and her late husband had another visit. The swelling in her legs subsided again after our session, just like it would after her massage that she would receive in the next week.

Once, as we were talking before she got on the table, she asked rather sharply:

"Why does my husband only come to visit me when you are here?"

I was a little taken back; I blurted out, "Because this is the only time you aren't busy." She appeared satisfied with the answer, and we began the session.

The last week I saw her, the wounds in her abdomen were pretty advanced. I could smell them. She was tired and not as energetic as before, but still in good spirits. We had a totally peaceful, physically grounding healing session: no fireworks, no visitors, no roller coaster. I could not turn her over because of the open lesions, so once again there was no Lymphatic Drain.

She died peacefully the following week.

Jane taught me to let go of my agenda and follow the energy. I had experienced a much greater intelligence than my own. It took me many, many healings before I learned to trust this intelligence with my whole being.

5

LETTING GO OF THE OUTCOME

I WORKED WITH A WOMAN WHO WAS RECOVERING FROM A life-threatening autoimmune disease. When she first came to see me, she had already healed herself from the most debilitating symptoms of the condition. She was not entirely back to normal and her recovery had plateaued. She still felt fatigued and emotionally drained most of the time.

For the first five or six healings, she made steady progress. She had more energy and started working part-time. It was very satisfying to hear about her improvement each week.

Then it seemed she plateaued again. She came for her healing every week, but when I checked in with her progress, there was not much obvious outward improvement, physically or emotionally, in her life.

At that time, I was very attached to helping my clients feel better, do better, be better. I had a very rigid idea of how my clients should heal. My mission as an energetic healer was to create healing, balance and improve people's quality of life. I was getting paid to make a difference and was very attached to her recovery.

I was lying awake at night asking myself: Was I really helping her? Was it ethical to keep taking her money every week when there was no discernible improvement? Should I say something?

She appeared happy to see me every week and enjoyed her time on the table. The sessions were extremely peaceful and calming.

Finally, after one of her sessions, I could not keep myself from asking: "What are you getting out of these healings?"

I will never forget her answer. The tone of her voice hit me as if a gong was struck inside my body. She said, "This is the only place I can relax."

I felt a wave of emotion reverberate through me as she spoke those words. I can't tell you how many clients tell me after a session how deeply relaxed they are, as if they had never felt it before. I realized the greatest gift I can give my client is a space for them to relax. When a body deeply relaxes, everything resets, restores and rebalances. A relaxed body heals itself. All healing is self-healing.

I was also noticing that in many of my sessions, I often felt my clients "click" into alignment. Like their nervous system suddenly reset. I realized creating a space for my clients to relax their nervous system was more important than the issues (headache, stress, fatigue) they had originally booked their appointment to heal.

Matt Kahn writes a lot about calming the nervous system. Here is one of my favorite quotes:

"Underneath it all, I came to discover that the source of a closed heart, a noisy mind, low self-esteem, or an out-of-control-ego is an overstimulated nervous system."

— MATT KAHN FROM HIS
BOOK *WHATEVER ARISES, LOVE THAT*

I vowed never to question the value of energy work again, no matter what the apparent outcome.

6

LETTING GO OF CONCEPTS AND TRAININGS

I HAVE FOUND THAT MY OWN IDEAS AND MENTAL CONCEPTS about the nature of energy have often been the very obstacles that keep me from directly experiencing what is actually happening in the healing session.

One idea of how the energy may be supporting one client often becomes the very block that prevents me from staying fully present for another client.

As my awareness of energy grew, outdated models and theories had to be thrown out.

Really, it's important to stay present with what is actually happening in the session as it happens. There are times when holding someone's feet with an intention to rebalance their energy can significantly reduce lower back pain, and there are times when holding the client's feet too intensely can give them a slight headache.

You would think that being a healer, that working daily in a profession so outside most conventional paradigms, I would naturally be more open-minded and flexible about things.

Wrong.

I found I held on tightly to my thoughts and philosophies of healing. Especially early on in my practice, I felt like I had to explain, even defend my ideas and the validity of my profession. The ideas that I felt I had to constantly defend made me more mentally rigid.

Being a professional energy healer is outside of most people's reality paradigm. I had a close friend from Texas who used to roll her eyes every time I said the word "chakra." As an energetic practitioner I had to get used to reactions like this outside the healing room. Yet, when I visited her after a minor operation, she asked me for a healing. I almost fell over.

How much I held on to my story of how energy worked became obvious to me during a workshop with Janna Moll, SEM, MSN, LMT, HTP in 2014 called "Advanced Chakra Diagnosis and Treatment."

Janna is a feisty Energy Medicine Instructor of twenty-five years. She is opinionated, honest, and tells it like it is. I learned quite a bit in that class.

Janna was working with a physicist and created a model of working with chakras as balls of energy instead of the cone-like shapes I had learned about in The Healing Touch Program. Since the start of my healing practice, I had been visualizing and working with the energy centers as cones like the ones that were illustrated in the book *Hands of Light* by Barbara Brennan. *Hands of Light* is still sacred to me; it was one of the first books about energy healing I had read.

During this workshop, Janna calmly starts telling the class how the chakras are really balls of energy instead of the cones. Janna was about to move to another subject—

as if she hadn't just blown my mind—when I raised my hand to extend the discussion. I found these ideas very, *very* upsetting. Very upsetting because I had a feeling she was right.

How could I be using the "wrong" model of the main energy centers and be getting such beneficial results for my clients? How could I have not known this? How could I just change how I work with energy?

I was obviously very attached to my ideas. Were my ideas blocking true perception? My brain hurt.

I somehow got over myself and started using the chakra ball concept in the workshop when I used the pendulum to access my client's energy. It worked well, even better than the cone concept when it came to hand placements. I could leave my elbows on the table and hold the first chakra and hips without the shoulder fatigue that came from holding my hands above the client's body. That helped me focus more. I switched to the ball model of energy work by the end of the workshop.

Yet, I was devastated and confused for weeks. How could I trust any conceptual model after such a mistake? How could I trust my perception of what was happening?

Then I just got used to being devastated. And I kept on doing healing work.

Now in my sessions, the energy shows up in the most accessible form for me to serve my client. Sometimes I even sense my client's energy in my old concept of the cone shaped chakras. I find this slightly nostalgic. Sometimes energy is a particle, sometimes a wave, sometimes everything, and sometimes energy feels like nothing— just stillness.

All the techniques I have learned over the years often still serve me when they arise in a session. Sometimes I sense the need to do a Mind Clearing from my initial Healing Touch Training, so then I do the sequence of hand positions for a Mind Clearing.

I usually do a Chakra Connection in my sessions; that series of hand placements from the feet to the head that balance and opens the whole energetic body. There are even times when I sense all I have to do is hold the space without even touching my client's body; just meditating close by brings everything into balance.

7

LETTING GO OF THE THOUGHT THAT I SHOULD NOT BE HAVING THOUGHTS

THIS IS DEFINITELY SOMETHING THAT TOOK ME YEARS TO come to terms with. If you struggle with an overactive brain, I hope this story and what I learned deepens your energy practice as much as it has mine. Letting go of the thought that I should not be having thoughts in my healing sessions was one of the most difficult blocks I had to detach from in order to completely trust the energy.

Most of the time there are no thoughts during a session. When thoughts do appear I have learned not to resist them; that they can even give me valuable insights into my client's healing process.

Many years ago I began a session with a new client, and as soon as I touched her leg, I instantly started having thoughts about my own childhood. I started thinking about how much I had longed for a dog when my family lived in a place that did not allow pets.

I was very judgmental about these thoughts. Why was I thinking about myself and my childhood? Why was I not focusing on the healing session, the client, and experiencing the healing compassion of sacred space? My thoughts were stressing me out.

When the session was over, despite my mental conflict, the client was elated. She shared with me how much she had been *longing* for the relationship that had just ended before she came for her healing. She had finally realized in the session that even though her heart had been broken when her boyfriend had recently left her, he was not the partner she really needed in her life. The *longing* she had been carrying for months was gone. She told me how clear, grounded, and grateful she now felt. A great weight had been lifted.

Every time she said the word "*longing*" I felt goose bumps on my arms. I realized this was the exact energy, the exact emotion, that came up for me when I had thoughts about not having a dog. My thoughts had obviously connected me to her healing process. The thoughts were a part of her session. I was amazed.

> *I would like to point out that even though "I" was thinking personal thoughts around this energy of longing during the session, "I" was not emotionally experiencing longing, like I had as a child.*
>
> *It's difficult to describe. Kind of like a kinesthetic awareness of a cloud floating by in the sky, except I am both the cloud, and the sky, and the observer all at once.*

There are still times when I begin a healing, in which my brain starts firing off like the 4th of July. This can happen even when everything else in the session feels completely still, and sometimes not. There is so much stimulating mental energy and monkey mind in the healing space that sometimes I even see little sparks around my eyes. When this happens, I know whoever I am working with is rebalancing some intense mental energy and I am experiencing a direct connection to it. This connection makes it easier for me to hold, channel, and just be present in the sacred healing space for as long as is necessary. The thoughts do not cause me stress anymore and there seem to be a lot less of them.

Sometimes during a healing I start thinking about something I watched on Netflix the night before, or a dream I had, or a comment a friend made. I notice all awarenesses around the thoughts: emotions like revenge, fear, grief, even romantic and nostalgic energies.

I notice body sensations: Is my stomach slightly nauseated (detox), do I feel warm, chilled, stiff, or has my breathing changed? I sometimes bring these observations up with the client, depending on the client and if I think anything I have to say may be helpful.

I ultimately use the thoughts to help me stay focused, grounded and present in the session. Then, of course there are times when there is helpful information for my client that has come in as a thought. Nothing is ever written in stone and every session is different.

Resistance to thoughts while in sacred space caused me much more stress than the thoughts themselves. When I let go of the thought that I should not be thinking, my ability to hold a clear healing vibration for my client became exponentially stronger.

8

SELF-JUDGMENT AND THE ENERGY OF ADDICTION

ONCE I WAS WORKING WITH A THERAPIST WHO HAD suddenly lost her job. She had recently moved to California specifically for this job, and so she did not have a supportive community around her during this upheaval in her life. In her third session, she had an emotional release around issues with her mother. She was crying and shaking on the table; the release took quite a while.

I sensed a "staleness" to her movements; something felt off. I initially labeled my observations as a judgment. A judgment because I am a big fan of crying. Crying is a great method of emotional release.

As I held the space for her to release, I felt an impulse to pass my open hand about six inches over her abdomen. I felt an energy that was so seductive my whole body relaxed. It was not sexual, yet it had a pull that was almost magnetic. I felt the urge to just lean over into the energy and fall into it.

I thought for sure I was imagining it, so I removed my

hand, re-grounded my own energy field, and then slowly passed my hand over her third chakra. Again, I felt the same sensations. Each time, it felt so tangible, irresistible, enticing.

I realized this was the energy of addiction. This woman was addicted to this story.

This was a powerful energy. I instantly had a whole new respect for addicts and all addictions.

After feeling it just this one time, I felt like I was already addicted to it. The root of my client's issue was the addiction to her story of being a victim in her relationship with her mother. She was enjoying her expression of it on my table.

I asked myself: What is the most healing thing I could say about this with my client? How can I bring this up with her in a way she could hear?

I did not address the addiction energy with my client at the end of this session. I just did not know what to say or how to say it. Unfortunately, this client found another job in another state and I did not get to work with her again. Her "stress" was over and she felt she did not need any more sessions.

After twenty more years of healings, I know these insights are a profound clue to helping my clients heal. Usually I don't have to bring anything up. In a few sessions the clients themselves become aware of what they need to address and release. I have found becoming conscious and aware of whatever is holding us back from being balanced and grounded is the healing. What we are conscious of cannot sabotage us. Just holding a nonjudgmental, healing presence is the most healing.

This was a profoundly helpful insight for me as an energetic healer and another lesson in learning to stay present with my client's process and trust my intuition.

9

LETTING GO OF THE DESIRE TO SEE AURAS

I HAD ALWAYS WANTED TO SEE THE AURAS OF MY CLIENTS. I mean physically "see" the colors, chakras, and energy flow of the biofield. I had read about other healers who could see auras, so when I first started my healing practice I thought that I would be a better healer if I could see the energy. I really wanted to be the best healer I could be.

So for the first ten years of my Healing Touch practice, I focused my eyes on the energy field of every person I worked with hoping that someday I would finally "see." I studied the Barbara Brennan books and illustrations, I meditated with the book *The Chakras* by C. W. Leadbeater, and I studied every other energy book I could find. I read about other people's experiences of seeing and opening up to the energy. I also painted my healing room a light blue, because I noticed that color seemed to visually bring out more activity around my client's heads (which it did.) I have always been able to sense and see activity close to the body that looks like a mirage in the desert—wavy or sparkly clear energy. I was obsessed.

Then finally, one day in 2010, I was looking at the illustrations in the book *The Path of The Dream Healer*. Adam McLeod's illustrations of auras showed human bodies surrounded by soft, glowing colors. I could always see that in my client's energy field.

Instantly I realized I had been seeing energy fields all along. What I had been expecting to see were the illustrations in the Barbara Brennan books and not really perceiving what was really in front of me. It was another one of those incredible "ah-ha" moments. I could now see auras and even show other people how to see auras too. It was so profound for me it felt a little surreal. I felt a little off and slightly ungrounded for a few days.

Again I found myself asking, What else was I not perceiving? What other ideas do I have about my healing practice that block me from experiencing what is actually happening?

I also found that learning to see auras did not make me a better healer. I still primarily get information about my client's energy by feeling their aura with my hands and by just "knowing" what I need to do in the session. Dropping my fixation with seeing auras felt like I had let go of a twenty-pound weight. It was liberating. It was getting easier to see what was actually helping me as a healer.

10

ENERGY AND SPIRIT GUIDES

I moved to San Francisco in 1988. I had gone to college in Denver, completed graduate school in Chicago, and now it was time to learn to meditate. I had a list. Meditation was the last box to check.

At this time I was working in the video industry as an editing house scheduler; a skill that became extremely useful when I started my own business.

I thought of myself as an artist. I was constantly making pinhole photographs, building my own cameras and printing black and white collage images based on the subtle energy body. My subject matter included images of auras, chakras, spirit guides, as well as crystals, X-rays, anatomy texts from books, and acupuncture needles.

Healing imagery had always fascinated me. I had no idea at that point that one day I would actually be studying in massage school, and later in my healing practice, the same books I was making art with.

When I arrived in San Francisco, I visited a few meditation schools to explore the different meditation styles and what was available. I went to one open house at a school where you sat in a circle facing the center with your eyes closed. Someone walked around the outer edge and every fifteen minutes or so slapped two boards together over your head to "wake you up." I did not find that school appealing.

I decided on a mediation school called Psychic Horizons. They talked about meditation as an accessible bridge between spirit and everyday life. Psychic Horizons sounded so practical and straight-forward. After the first three seven-week classes I took the Clairvoyant training, which was a lot more than just practical. It was one of the best things I have ever done. This was an incredible adventure in which I learned what it was like to be grounded, run energy through my physical body, and do energy readings for others. I also began to work with spirit guides.

I was not a natural at working with spirit guides. I felt I actually failed spirit guide class. When my group closed our eyes and were guided through a process of being introduced to our "Healing Master" I just didn't get it. I even opened my eyes to see if anyone else was having a problem. It seemed to me the rest of the class seemed to have gotten it. I was about a week behind after that. I felt like I was just imagining any guides I might be connecting with. I never really believed or trusted the whole "spirit guide" concept, even though I really admired the other meditators who seem to receive so much valuable information from their guides.

I started my massage practice about five years after graduating from Psychic Horizons. Yet, I had picked up the idea in massage school that psychically "reading" my client's energy was a violation of my client's privacy. I was a massage therapist, not a psychic reader. These are the kinds of ideas that can really hold you back when working with energy. I was blocking my ability to "read" my client's energetic field right from the start when I opened my business. Yet, who knows? Maybe that helped me focus.

Anyway, I learned a lot about energy as a Massage Therapist.

Steve was one of my first massage clients. He was a charming, good-looking guy with a bit of a wild side.

At the start of his first massage, as soon as my hands touched his back, I sensed something extra in the room. About twenty minutes into the massage I felt the unmistakable presence of two beings at the table. As I finished massaging his back, I moved from the top of the table to his right arm. I walked the long way around the table because there was something, or someone, just off to my right, by his shoulder. I had no idea what to do.

What was going on? Was this good? Was this not so good?

I decided I had to ask myself what I felt.

I felt that there was only positive energy in the room. That was comforting. I continued with the massage.

Even though my brain was freaking out trying to process all the ramifications of what was happening, I stayed focused on the session and confirmed that there were at least two very loving, tangible presences in the room. By the end of the session, one was on each side of the table. I had never felt such a solid presence of "other" energy before. These were not imaginary spirits. I could really feel them. Experiencing this just changed things for me on a very practical, tangible level.

There really are spirit guides, angels, or whatever these presences were. They exist in this reality. I was now a believer.

They also seemed to have nothing to convey to me. Which was fine with me. They were there to connect with Steve. All good.

At the end of the session I walked into the other room and started writing my notes about the massage while Steve got off the table and dressed. He walks in and tells me how much he liked the massage. He was so surprised to feel me working on two or three places at the same time; he felt me holding his hand while at the same time massaging his leg.

I had no idea how to respond.

I can't remember what I said that first session, but I know I told him I was glad he liked the massage. In subsequent sessions, he always had spirit guides and other beings around him and every massage revealed to me a new level of surrender to the healing possibilities of the massage space. I started telling him about my experiences during the massages and we started talking about other mystical experiences in his life. He began to open up to his intuitive abilities and started to trust them. We both learned a lot while working together.

It was incredibly interesting. He crashed his motorcycle a few times and lived a pretty exciting life. I always wondered why he had so many loving guides around him. We worked together for several years until he moved to the East Coast.

For me, I had begun to learn to trust what was

happening in my sessions no matter what my previous beliefs had been. I had to acknowledge that there were beings without bodies. Of course, what choice did I have? Pretend it wasn't happening? I was always fascinated by the ideas of spirit guides, guardian angels, even though I had never tangibly believed that they existed. Now I was open to that reality on a whole new level. I developed much deeper levels of trust working with this one client alone. My concept of reality was opening up in a big way. It was very exciting.

Working with spirit guides is not one of my gifts, Yet, they show up in my healing sessions in different ways to connect with my clients. Energy shows up as spirit guides, angels, deceased family members, spiritual teachers, power animals, avatars—whatever best serves my client in their healing. They move energy, bring in energy, and sometimes communicate directly with the person on the table. They are extremely powerful allies in the healing space.

I use invocations before almost every healing session; I always "call in" or "open this moment to the invisible realms" to invite helpful spirits and allies in. I find speaking the intentions I have just discussed before the healing with my clients very powerful.

I would like to note here I have not had any problem with "bad" energy or unhelpful spirits. I think this may be one of my inherent abilities—to hold a safe, grounded healing space. I have never had to protect myself or my clients. I sense "bad" energy as stuck memories, emotions, and areas where the energy is congested. I hold a high vibration (different for every client and every session) where anything of a lower vibration has to leave.

I have felt some "falling away of energy" that has been extremely 'dramatic' in my sessions. I am sure entities have been released, past lives resolved, and soul retrievals facilitated in my client's healings, yet I have found it is not important to label all that happens. I also hold everything in sacred space with great respect, even that which falls away.

We humans have so much more help available to us than we ever dreamed possible. We just have to trust it.

11

MIGRAINES AND THE INCLUSIVE
HEALING NATURE OF SACRED SPACE

I FIRST LEARNED ABOUT THE INCLUSIVE HEALING POWER OF the sacred space because of my migraines. I didn't realize this when it was happening. As I began to look back and connect the dots, this was where I learned the skill of paying attention to and holding space for my body as well as my client's body, and eventually everything else in the room.

When I began my healing practice as a massage therapist I had horrible, debilitating, recurring migraines. I had these headaches for about thirteen years and I remember them getting worse in massage school. I discovered Clarity Breathwork in 2006 and healed myself that year. (I write more about how I healed my migraines with Clarity Breathwork in Chapter 30, " Clarity Breathwork.")

The migraines frequently started with the right side of my body feeling tighter than my left, and then a horrendous pounding developed in my head, sometimes my sinuses. A full blown headache would last three days, often resulting in a long stretch of projectile vomiting. I vividly remember one day in which I was lying on the floor in so much pain, I thought if I didn't know this was only going to last three days I would go crazy. I learned a lot about the nature of pain during this time.

In the last year of being sick, I had some form of a headache every weekend. I stopped going to weekend workshops because I would always be sick. The migraines had taken over my life.

There were so many workdays in which I would wake up with a headache that was about a five on a scale of one through ten. If I was not throwing up I would work. I worked because I wanted to work. I loved my work. In thirteen years I very seldom cancelled my clients. I write more about this in Chapter 31, "Checking In—Should I Work Today?"

I discovered right away that when I was actually giving a massage when I had a headache, the pain would become much less intense. A few minutes into the first session of the day I would always feel significantly better. At the end of the day I always felt so much better than when I started the workday.

While I was giving a massage and totally focused on my client, I was also aware of the throbbing pain in my head. I developed a dual awareness of my body and energy, as well as my client's. My migraine would always ease up about ten minutes into the session and return about ten minutes after the session ended. The headache was always much less intense after each session.

Only years later did I realize what the migraines had taught me. They trained me to develop a dual awareness in the healing space, and that I am just as much a part of the healing as my clients are.

There was a belief floating around in the Healing Touch Community during the years I was being certified, that if the practitioner was sick, the energy would go to the healer instead of the healee. I always felt really bad about this and thought because I had a low grade headache my client would receive less energy. Yet, I learned this is just not the case for me. My clients had powerful healings and heart opening sessions whether I had a headache or not. It took me years to let go of that belief.

There is so much energy available to us. The healing space can hold everything and heal everything that is ready to be healed.

12

LETTING GO OF THE SPIRITUAL SEEKER

FOR THE FIRST TWENTY YEARS OF MY HEALING PRACTICE, MY spiritual seeking and my healing work were the same thing.

Now they are not.

I used to be very excited about achieving a higher state of consciousness in my healing sessions. Now my life is about being present in this moment, right here and right now, as I spell check these words.

I found the portal to all possibilities is in the present moment, not in an altered state of consciousness. At this point I would say that altered states of consciousness that help us heal are multidimensional aspects of this moment. It's all right here.

Letting go of the spiritual seeker took about seven years. Seven grueling years. It was one of those "dark night of the soul" things. It was exhausting, unnecessary, and even a little embarrassing while I was going through it.

My healing practice now is about being in service to others. It's also about making a living.

Having to earn a living made me address every obstacle that appeared in my healing practice, not give up when things became confusing. When I have to work I have to stay focused. This is why having a healing business has been such a gift for me and why I would like to encourage others in their practice. If I didn't have to make a living I might not have continued when things started falling apart—or what I thought was falling apart.

It's also important to state here that all healing practices are valuable, whether you make a living or not. Exploring energetic healing to primarily heal yourself and your family and friends is the most powerful thing you can do for yourself and the world. You can open up abilities in yourself that can make a difference in every aspect of your life: your business, your relationships, your health.

I had been a spiritual seeker before I even knew what a spiritual seeker was. When I was a child I was driven to find out how the world worked. What I had observed about life just did not make sense; we are born, grow up, grow old, and then die. Something seemed to be missing. It was a game that didn't seem worth playing.

13

THE SPIRITUAL IN ART

I STUDIED ART IN COLLEGE AND FOUND THE ACT OF creating took me beyond what I thought was mundane reality and allowed me to touch that "thing," that "truth" beyond the surface. Studying ceramics, photography and video, I found I connected with the work of artists like Diane Arbus, Minor White, Ralph Eugene Meatyard, Maya Deren, and Morris Graves.

After graduate school at the Art Institute of Chicago, I worked in the video industry, and taught photography, video, and art in the San Francisco Bay Area for about ten years. I decided (rather abruptly right after having my taxes done in 1995), that I was not going to be able to support myself as a professional artist or teacher. This was a rude awakening, an ego crash, an unmistakable fork in the road.

I had to make a living. So what was the one thing I was interested in besides art? Massage. I always loved massage. So I went to massage school. At the time a career change like this probably appeared to my friends to be one of the most absurd things I could have done. I was thirty-five, which seemed a little late to begin the physical profession of massage. My whole life was about making art, and I was way, way, way, in debt. Thank God I had supportive friends.

The massage school debt was added to the art school debt, and I was very financially motivated to make my massage practice work. Financial limitation is a tangible boundary, and clear boundaries made manifestation possible. I found lack of finances can be grounding.

Having a massage and healing business was also a gift for me, because it kept that edge between practical and woo-woo very sharp. I was in a business support group for two years and my tagline every week was "Jeri Lawson, Healing Touch Practitioner. It's not woo-woo if it works."

The polarity between money and energy is a great teacher. Having a healing business is like a constant walk between worlds.

It felt so good to help other people feel better. Then from 2001 to 2013, I found great satisfaction in bringing energetic work into my established massage practice and holding higher states of consciousness on a daily basis. My practice focused on energetically supporting people through chemotherapy and radiation.

I thought I would become "enlightened" from being in elevated energetic states five days a week. Even though my massage sessions brought me to a place of focus, presence, and higher frequencies of energy, Healing Touch and Reiki appeared to be a direct route to waking up from ego and transcending habitual, mundane, reality. I was still a Type A spiritual seeker, on a fascinating wild ride, and every session brought me closer to enlightenment, nirvana, liberation of the ego, and truth-realization. I had a focus, a mission, a purpose.

All through these years my energetic healing practice was also profoundly helping my clients as my massage practice had: alleviating emotional and physical pain, supporting people through chemotherapy, radiation, addiction, divorce, and many times connecting them with their highest guidance and wisdom. I was also earning a living, paying my mortgage, and looking forward to every day of work. I was highly motivated and learning with every session how to be the best healer I could be. I was living the dream.

Then, 2013 was about the time I realized I was not using many of the techniques I had learned in my Healing Touch training. I was still diagnosing my client's energy with my hands and pendulum as taught in the Healing Touch Training Program, yet I was mostly only doing a long Chakra connection in my sessions.

After the chakra connection, when I checked my client's energy field, it had come into balance without the use of other techniques. This was good, because after the Chakra Connection I didn't have any time left in the session. I didn't know it yet, but I was already holding space for the client to heal themselves. I was letting go of my Healing Touch Training and following the energy. I found this stressful, because Healing Touch had been the foundation of my healing practice and had served me well.

14

THE BOOK

THIS WAS WHEN I READ *SPIRITUAL ENLIGHTENMENT: THE Damnedest Thing.* This book introduced me to the concept of non-duality and initiated the seven year process that eventually brought all my spiritual seeking outside myself to a close. This was the beginning of the end of my exhilarating spiritual journey.

Spiritual Enlightenment: The Damnedest Thing is narrated by a fictional character named Jed McKenna. Jed McKenna is a man who realized the non-dual state in his 20s. He is a kind of spiritual teacher in a rural area of the Midwest. He describes himself as someone "not really able to form attachments with adult humans."

I do not recommend reading this book unless you just can't help yourself. There are easier introductions to finding unity consciousness and realizing truth. Just saying.

I reread *Spiritual Enlightenment: The Damnedest Thing* while writing this book, just to be able to review all that it activated in my life. I can see now that there is another way to be in the world, be truth-realized, and awaken from the "dream," as described in this book. It's how the character Sonaya lives in the world. Jed writes a little over one page describing this fictional character, a woman who runs the house at his school.

Sonaya had been with the International Society for Krishna Consciousness for about twenty-five years before meeting Jed. Her devotion was to her Lord Krishna. She had explained to Jed that when she was with the Society she wasn't really with them; she was with Krishna. When she was with Jed, she wasn't with Jed; she was with Krishna.

Jed writes, "...eventually I realized that in all things, in every action, in every second of every day, she was practicing a conscious devotion to her Lord. It might look like she was cooking for the group or washing the floors for her own sense of cleanliness or managing the complexities of a diverse group of people for the benefit of those people or running an accidental ashram for me, but once I got the hang of her and really started paying attention to the way she paid attention to, well, everything, then I saw it. She was present in every moment, and every moment was a devotion to Lord Krishna."

After reading *Spiritual Enlightenment,* I now had an intellectual understanding of non-duality. I knew on a very deep level this was the truth that I had been searching for my entire life, even though it was not my current experience.

I found this whole revelation incredibly, profoundly disappointing. Heartbreaking, really. There was no bliss, no perfection, no ecstasy. The extraordinary turned out to be the most ordinary. I don't think I could even grasp the emotional impact of this when it happened, hence the seven year integration.

Throughout my life up to that point, my internal compass had been based in emotion and egoic desire, and now that compass, that way of being in the world, was gone. I had no direction. I couldn't feel anything. I had no idea what was important or worthwhile anymore.

What was even interesting? What the hell was happening? Was this a midlife crisis? Was this some kind biological process that everyone went through when they reached their 50s and found that nothing means anything?

What was once thrilling to me was gone. Like walking into a metaphysical bookstore and searching for that next book or idea that would open the great gates of higher consciousness. Like taking that next workshop or studying with the next great teacher. I missed the thrill of the hunt for something outside myself. I missed having a purpose.

Joan sums up what I discovered:

"I used to think enlightenment meant crossing some magical finish-line and living forever in a state of perfection and perpetual happiness. But enlightenment isn't about becoming perfect, I discovered, of finally getting control of my life and fixing it all up at last. The whole search for perfection and future happiness turns out to be a kind of distraction that obscures the realization that this moment already is the Holy Reality."

— JOAN TOLLIFSON IN *DEATH: THE END*
OF SELF-IMPROVEMENT, PAGE 27-28

I reread many of my spiritual books by Rupert Spira, Adyashanti, Eckart Tolle, Tony Parsons, Joan Tollifson, Gangaji, Richard Sylvester, and Darryl Bailey. I reread *The Course of Miracles* and it finally began to make sense. I also listened to awakening consciousness stories of ordinary people from Buddha at the Gas Pump, which is a huge resource. Rich Archer is one of my all-time heroes.

I realized this idea of oneness, this concept of non-duality, was what was being described all along in everyplace I looked. Nothing outwardly changed. I kept going through the motions of everyday life, but it was all different. After a while I just got used to it. Eventually there was nothing left but a deep dissatisfaction, or grief, and even that eventually disappeared.

My healing practice, which still included massage, continued on despite my spiritual crisis. I had to make a living and the sessions were obviously still very powerful for my clients. I was really making a difference in people's lives who were in physical pain, healing from cancer, or coping with anxiety. That was still satisfying and very grounding for me, even though I now felt like a spiritual imposter.

15

ANIMAL REIKI

THEN EVERYTHING BEGAN TO TURN AROUND. ON FACEBOOK, I discovered Kathleen Prasad's videos on Animal Reiki. Here was this woman who looked like she was about twelve, talking clearly and intelligently about "Being Reiki" rather than "Doing Reiki." She talked about creating an energetic healing space around yourself and letting the animals decide how much healing or time they needed in this space. When the animals knew they had enough, they just walked away.

I started studying with Kathleen and found her animal healing philosophy mirrored my own experience with people. I can't tell you how grateful I was, and still am, for Kathleen's teachings. She now developed a new method of animal-guided healing and meditation called Let Animals Lead®.

Working with Kathleen, and later her teacher Frans Stiene, I felt that the path my healing practice had taken started to make more sense. I really didn't need the techniques and hand positions I had learned in my Healing

Touch training. It was not necessary to even touch my client to create a space of profound healing for them. Instead of "giving" healing energy. I was "being" healing energy.

I started to let go of my need to know why the sessions were so effective, or not effective. I was so relieved. The spiritual seeker continued to fall away. I bought about 100 copies of *Reiki For Dogs* and gave everyone I met a copy, especially when I was walking my dog Berkeley. It is a brilliant meditation and healing book.

I had finally aligned my healing practice, my studies in non-duality, and even my love for animals, with the underlying principles of Animal Reiki.

16

ANIMAL REIKI BECOMES PEOPLE REIKI

THE DAY AFTER, LIKE THE FOLLOWING MONDAY AFTER I completed Kathleen Prasad's Reiki III and Animal Reiki Teacher Training workshop, one of my regular clients ended up in one of the nearby hospitals with an acute case of sepsis.

She had a cyst removed as an outpatient at the doctor's office. A few hours later she had a life-threatening infection. Her friend, who is also one of my clients, had called to let me know what was happening and where she was.

The universe had lined everything up for me to be able to go to the hospital in the middle of that afternoon. I had two back-to-back cancellations the day before and had a four-hour spot in the middle of the day. This type of sudden opening in my schedule has happened several times before when I needed to be somewhere else besides in my office. I am always still astounded at the synchronicity. You would think I would get used to it by now, but it still throws me sometimes. The world is so connected.

When I got to the hospital, it was obvious how serious the situation was. Sepsis is a serious condition of harmful microorganisms in the blood. The body's response to these microorganisms can potentially lead to the malfunctioning of organs, shock, and even death.

She barely knew I was there. I did a Healing Touch session, which balanced her energy and allowed her to fall into a deeply relaxed state.

After the session was over, there was no one in the room except the two of us. I did not want to leave her alone, so until another family member arrived, I sat by her bed. I realized I had started doing the Joshin Kokyu Ho meditation that I had just learned in my Animal Reiki workshop.

So I went with it. I was breathing into my hara, or lower belly, and on the exhale, expanding the energy out all around me and into the room, creating a healing space. This is a simple meditation technique that is in Kathleen's book *Reiki For Dogs,* page 31. I highly recommend this book.

The room changed in a matter of three deep breaths. There was *so much* energy, and in that energy everything was alive. The room was very bright, almost sparkly white. My client started having gentle muscle spasms throughout her body and appeared to be in communication with someone, or something I couldn't see. It felt like a spontaneous crack between worlds.

It was powerful. I felt like a bystander. I just held the space, stayed grounded and upright, and kept breathing.

It was just crazy; I had no context for what was happening.

Finally, the energy subsided. I really don't remember how long it lasted. There was no sense of time. Yet, when I left I knew she was going to be okay.

She completely recovered.

When I checked in with my client a week after, she said she remembered me coming to the hospital and that the healing was the point where "everything turned around."

I emailed her many years after to ask permission to tell her story in one of my blog posts. I had not shared my experience of the session with her before this. She replied:

> *"Wonderful to read your thoughts and description of what was for me an incomprehensible experience that just left me with an overall sense of well-being... I just know that I remember little fleeting things, like you coming into the room, your hands above me in the bed, a nurse poking her head into the room and your glance at her after which she simply nodded, turned, and left... closing the door. I felt utterly and totally relaxed and I distinctly remember "calming down." I distinctly remember feeling that you were in control of the room. (Why had the the nurse left?!)"*

Let me say right away I was not in control of anything. Once again, the less control I feel I have, the more profound the healing for my client. The nurse saw what I was doing and gave me the space to do it.

17

REDEFINING COMPASSION AND THE LIVING FLUID INTELLIGENCE

MY NEXT BIG CONCEPTUAL HURDLE WAS THE DILEMMA I HAD about compassion. I would like to write about it because it was such an issue with me for so long. I don't think this compassion issue is a rite of passage that every healer will go through, yet working with energy means you will probably go through something. Maybe how I navigated my something will help you with your something.

I kept reading about healers who were describing the healing space as heart-centered, bliss-filled, and compassionate. The thought that I was not experiencing compassion in the healing space was one of my great stumbling blocks in surrendering to the direct experience of healing for a long time. I felt like I was missing the boat. I was not feeling compassion in the healing space. I felt almost everything else, but not an all-consuming, heart-opening, compassionate emotion. Was I burnt out?

I finally found a description of the healing space that made a lot of sense to me. In Adyashanti's *The Way Of Liberation*, Adya writes about the Inner Revolution, the process that happens after the discovery of one's true nature. He describes this inner revolution as "the birth of a living, fluid intelligence."

A Living, Fluid Intelligence. That is exactly what I experience in the sacred healing space. A continually changing, evolving energy that is different every time, for every person. I had not had an inner revolution yet, and I do not live in my true nature all the time. When I am not in a healing session, I still feel most often like I am a physical body in the world.

Yet, I found the description of a living fluid intelligence very comforting and the perfect description of how energy moves in a healing. The drive to find the right words to describe and communicate what was happening in my healing practice was a very important part of understanding the nature of healing. It was important until it wasn't important.

18

FRANS STIENE

ONE OF THE MOST BRILLIANT HEALING AND enlightenment teachers I have ever studied with is Frans Stiene from the International House of Reiki. Frans was a teacher of Kathleen Prasad, the founder of Animal Reiki. His teachings and workshops were profoundly helpful for me to further understand my direct experiences of the healing space and of my life. If Frans is teaching in your area, I highly recommend his classes.

The desire and agenda to help others feel better was falling away, which ultimately made me a more effective healer. This desire had been my motivation and internal guide in my work and my life, and now I felt so much less ambitious in general, which was very uncomfortable and depressing. Just being in the world was now requiring a new method of navigation that was so confusing. There was much less ego. This was stressful. This was a big part of my dark night of the soul.

Finally one Monday morning I had a little breakdown. I somewhat frantically whipped out an email to Frans:

Frans,

Do you use the word compassion, like other practitioners use the word love? Like everything is energy, reiki and love?

The word Compassion for me describes an emotional state, and the healing space for me is not emotional.

The best description I have found of the healing state is from Adayshanti's Way of Liberation book. He describes the "fluid living intelligence" that is experienced after an awakening. I am not "awake" but I certainly am in the Fluid Living Intelligence when I share Reiki with others.

Any thoughts?

Thanks,

Jeri

He emailed back right away. I just love this guy.

Hi Jeri,

For me compassion is not emotional at all.

True compassion is from a space of no giver, receiver and gift.

This is also why we can say love or true love, true love is like compassion, love can be contaminated by our confused mind.

But we all have to use words we like for that space.

For me fluid living intelligence is too wordy and too much in the head.

So find your way and your words.
Love
Frans

As soon as I read his email everything shifted.
Just. Like. That.
It really felt like Frans's response was an energetic transmission, a healing, because it was so instantaneous. My mind had certainly been confused. I will be forever grateful to Frans.

19

THE INTENSITY OF STILLNESS

THE WHOLE COMPASSION/DETACHMENT POLARITY CAME UP again in a series of emails I had with a client right after an intense emotional release in her healing. She often writes me about her experiences in our sessions in great detail a day or so after her session. I have learned so much from her writings. In this particular session, she shared with me that she had a huge emotional release while I had been in a completely nonemotional, detached state.

"It's fascinating how different our experiences are in the same session. So different—and yet, almost all the time, you are able to give me exactly what I need. I would certainly not wish the intensity of emotion I had on anyone (though I needed it)—and I think I needed you to have such calm so I could do what I needed. I am still feeling predominantly internally calm and grounded. Still intermittently anxious, but the anxiety is only in the background. It feels like a gift to be able to feel like my 'normal' self for a little while in this surreal world."

I wrote back:

"...When my clients have the most intense sessions—the most emotion, the most healing, the most physical sensations—I am usually the most 'detached' emotionally. It was so confusing for me for so long. I am holding the space for you to heal and rebalance. The space holds you."

She wrote:

"It does make sense, from a healing perspective at least, for you to have stillness as I experience the most intensity; it makes me wonder what would happen if your intensity matched mine; I wonder if the intensities and energies would cancel themselves out or not be able to hold each other if that were the case?"

I realized from our exchange that describing a state of consciousness as "detached" or "still" suggests there is no intensity.

Wrong.

I realized there is a profound intensity in the space I describe as still and detached. Dramatic emotional release is so obviously intense. The stillness is profoundly intense. It is unmatched.

Words are tricky.

20

BOREDOM AS A THRESHOLD

ONE DAY HEATHER CAME FOR A SESSION ABOUT FIVE YEARS after starting her full-time healing business. She was perplexed.

She told me she found herself feeling bored in her healings.

Heather is one of the most heart-centered, empathic, and caring people I have ever met. She is a very conscious mother of three very sensitive and self-aware daughters. She is a gifted healer and one of the most compassionate human beings on the planet. I am in awe of her abilities. If she feels bored, it is not from absence of motivation to help others, or lack of focus.

I knew exactly what she was experiencing.

I asked her to describe "bored."

She talked about feeling disconnected from her client, like nothing was happening under her hands. She had thoughts of "What am I doing?" "Nothing is happening here," and "This makes no sense anymore."

I suggested she go into the experience of "bored" with

great curiosity. Was it an internal experience? External? What was the physical sensation of being bored in her own body? What were the thoughts attached to this feeling/sensation? I encouraged her to explore the experience of being bored as you would any other energy. I proposed that boredom could be a portal into something much greater.

> *The experience of being bored or disconnected from your client can be a threshold to a great opening of consciousness. It may be that your client is bored or disconnected from their life. It could also be a lack of focus or a sign of you being burned out. It could be anything. Notice without judgment. It's just information. Be curious.*

I was very confused and judgmental when boredom showed up in my practice. This was at the beginning of that crazy seven-year stretch, when I noticed I was using less Healing Touch techniques, when I was worried I had lost my compassion, that I wondered if I was burned out, and when my desire to be the greatest healer possible started falling away. It was scary.

This was all part of my process of letting go of spiritual seeking. It also seemed that the more powerful and effective the healing space was becoming for my clients, the less emotionally attached I felt to the healing process.

All this drama was totally unnecessary. This is why I am writing this book. In one conversation Heather walked right through this whole mind melt. I wonder if other healers get to this place where they feel bored and detached and just stop working, thinking they are burned out.

Six months after our initial conversation Heather and I had another discussion about being bored. She had arrived at a whole new level of awareness that she said she would never have been able to understand before.

"Allowing myself to be a witness to what I was feeling and experiencing without judgment opened the door to higher consciousness and more profound sessions for my clients. After years of living with anxiety and depression, this new sense of peace and awareness I was experiencing was, in a way, unnerving. My mind, body, and soul were quiet and connected for perhaps the first time in my life. Not knowing what this feeling was, I confused it with boredom instead of content-ment, driven by universal support. I was content, fully present, connected, grounded, and open."

— HEATHER SWALLOW

Now I realize that this reality, the present moment is where everything exists—the past, the present, the future. It is the direct experience of this moment, the same moment you are reading these words, is where all the answers and all the questions are.

21

ALL POSSIBILITIES EXIST IN EVERY MOMENT—HOLDING SPACE FOR LIFE AND DEATH

FOR ME, THE PORTAL OF BOREDOM AND MY UNDERSTANDING of non-duality was the path to that place where all possibilities exist. For me, the emotionless, egoless state holds the ultimate healing for another human being.

I work with people who appear to be very "sick." They are often very stressed and even embarrassed from the pain they think they are causing the people they love.

As healer, just being able to hold a space for your client to acknowledge the possibility of their own death, of not getting "better," could be the exact thing that saves their life.

One of the first clients I energetically supported through chemotherapy was having a tough time. I would go to his home weekly, let myself in his house, and give him a healing session on his bed. He would be fast asleep when I was finished and I would let myself out without waking him.

He was physically very compromised. After many of

our sessions, I wondered if he would still be alive when I came back the following week. He was not looking good. His sister had initially called me in to see him, and even though these sessions were his first experience of energy work, he felt it was really helping him.

My brain kept racing into the future between visits. Is he going to die? Should I be doing more chakra spreads (a technique often used for transitions) rather than clearing techniques? I just kept following the energy through each individual session as if each session was the first time I had ever worked with him. During our healings everything felt "right." Yet, between sessions I was worried.

He fully recovered. When I see him now almost twenty years later he looks great. This was one of my first lessons in not judging the future in the present. The client may live or the client may not live, but they are alive right here, right now, and that is the only thing that is important.

In 2014 I worked with one of the most personally challenging clients I have ever had. She appeared to her community to be dying. She had cancer throughout her body, protruding lymph nodes in her groin, had several late-night ER visits, lost a huge amount of weight, and could barely walk. This woman was fully committed to having everyone who worked with her believe she was going to live. On my first visit she looked me straight in the eye and very aggressively asked, "Do you think I am going to die?"

I felt attacked. She had a very confrontational personality. The answer that came through my mouth was "all possibilities exist in this moment."

She nodded, satisfied, and we started our session. I have no idea where that response came from, but I felt like I had dodged a bullet. I dodged a lot of bullets with that client. I learned a lot from her and I chose to keep working with her, even though I had to schedule personal recovery time after every session. I highly respect her. She ended up fully healing herself and went back to work.

22

EXPLORING SACRED SPACE AND THE HEALING STATE

FROM 2014 TO 2019 I WENT THOUGH CHANGES ON EVERY level of my life and being. I had a massive, disruptive kundalini opening. It was horrible. My whole life changed; I got a divorce and moved out of my home. I did lose fourteen pounds, so that goes to show you there is always a silver lining.

I learned first-hand how powerful the non-judgmental healing space was when my Breathworker, Sophia Arise, held the space for my healing.

I was such a mess. I would go to my breath session with her and feel worse after the session. It was a very difficult year. I felt so much shame. Shame for getting into this situation and shame for not feeling better. Sophia held such a high space. She wasn't attached to me getting better; my "not" healing did not reflect on her abilities as a breathworker.

To be able to hold space for someone not to heal is a superpower.

She held a space for me that was completely without

judgment, with such grace. I realized first hand how profoundly healing it is to have someone hold this space for you.

This was truly where all possibilities, all healing, exists.

23

ISHAYA ASCENSION AND RETREAT
IN OCTOBER OF 2018

THIS CHAPTER IS ABOUT MY OWN EXPLORATIONS OF consciousness, separate from the healing space. I think it is important to write about these discoveries because this is when the spiritual seeking ended and my healing practice truly and completely became an act of service.

I met Neika Supriya Whittemore around 2014. My friend Mary Gaetjens and I had started doing Breathwork circles in Oakland, and Supriya came to support several of them.

We were just starting out facilitating circles together and her presence was very supportive. Supriya was so grounded and calm; she talked me off the ledge several times at the crucial beginning of my "dark night of the soul."

Talking with another person who could hold space for me in that period was extremely helpful when my ego was melting down. Especially when I didn't feel like I was even talking, it was more like whining on and on about something that I couldn't even describe.

I was so outwardly successful, living the dream as a full-time healer. The letting go of the spiritual seeker was devastating. I think this is why gurus are so popular.

I know I would have done anything to "understand" what was happening to me. I would have listened to anyone who even pretended like they knew the true nature of reality and what I was experiencing in this non-duality hell. We are so lucky to have the Internet and so many books about this process available now.

And I was lucky to have met Supriya. So I asked Supriya to be my meditation teacher in 2015. Supriya is an Ishaya Monk, and asking her to be my teacher was a big deal in the Ishaya world. I had no idea what an Ishaya was, but I had just asked to become a monk.

Ishaya is a Sanskrit word that means "for Christ-Consciousness" or "Enlightenment" The Ishaya ascension meditation is a set of simple mantra-like techniques which are based on Praise, Gratitude, Love, and Compassion. I took the initial class in May of 2015 and still practice daily. I find it grounding as consciousness, healing and life continues to unfold.

> *"Everything is in preparation to be unified with our Highest Self. We are all wired up for that. For those who have devoted their lives to that experience, there are practices that we can engage in to prepare for the union. To prepare our minds, central nervous system, relationships, and bodies for yoga—to sit in meditation effortlessly—and to remain there permanently. The sages say that life actually begins at that point of union. The invitation and opportunity is for you to have a direct experience of that in this lifetime. It's not*

a big deal. It is all simple and natural for each of us.
The Ishayas Ascension is our base. The Stillness is our
focus. What we put our attention on expands
effortlessly."

— SUPRYA ISHAYA

So I became an Ishaya Monk. Mentally it felt like a backward move. Here I am a student of non-duality and the present moment as a portal to the formless. Nevertheless, I found being in the small Universal Ishaya community of people focused on inner work is very nurturing to me. I found the rituals grounding.

Ascension, meditation, breathwork, and community calms my ego and my obsessive personality I still identify with. I found the pujas, Ascension techniques, and space of the month-long retreats incredibly valuable. Plus, I can bring my dog, Berkeley to the retreat. Berkeley eventually became Brighu, the little white Ishaya, since he went through my vows with me.

In 2018 I did a month long meditation retreat with my Ishaya community. One big question that I was constantly, obsessively asking myself before 2018 was: What is the nature of the healing space, the fluid living intelligence, as compared to the truth realization, liberation, the state of non-duality?

On the day my dog Berkeley and I started the retreat, there was a Supreme Court issue that greatly upset me. So when I sat to meditate my emotional body was quite activated. I was very angry. I could feel my energy spiraling and unwinding about five feet all around me, with waves of heat and nausea periodically passing through my physical body. It was very similar to the healing space I held for others, except I was feeling my own energy moving.

I would like to note here that my clients rarely feel nauseous.

For the first ten days, it was extremely challenging and physically uncomfortable to sit and meditate. I just wanted to run, to move, to get a drink of water, or find my cell phone and text for help.

Then I began to notice a space underneath all the movement. A quiet space. I focused on that, and it expanded over time and became more encompassing, eventually surrounding everything including my energy field and my body. My nervous system and energy field started settling down, and I experienced the heat and waves of nausea less and less.

This new space was utterly still, like a flat void. I could not even describe it as peaceful, certainly not compassionate, Yet, there was definitely no stress. It was empty of movement.

After ten days of emotional turmoil arising and releasing, this was a welcome shift. I focused on this space for the rest of my meditation retreat, and just let all my questions about healing states and consciousness go. In this space there is nothing to seek anymore. Everything is right here, in this stillness, in this emptiness.

What was most surprising is that even though this deeper space is still experienced as emotionally empty, I returned from the retreat feeling more compassion, joy, love, and clarity in all aspects of my life. I can listen to the daily news with much less resistance. I am less critical of myself. The more I connect with this space, the calmer and more peaceful I am.

You would think that connecting with a state of consciousness that creates more compassion would be experienced as compassionate. However, that's not how it works for me. The experience of emptiness in meditation created more compassion in my daily life, but I did not experience the emptiness as compassionate.

This discovery released my obsessive questioning of the healing space. I had let go of another level of needing to understand and control. It was a huge shift. It didn't matter to me what the nature of the fluid living intelligence was anymore: I found I even trusted it more deeply.

This is where I am at the moment in my healing practice and my life, and this moment is the only place I want to be. I do not sense that I am Awake with the big "A." I do feel that I am not seeking anymore, not looking outside myself for anything. It's a huge relief and very different.

24

THE VALUE OF LIVING IN
ENERGETIC ALIGNMENT: LIVING
DIFFERENTLY

WHEN MY CLIENTS RECEIVE A SERIES OF REIKI, HEALING
Touch and Breathwork sessions, it often changes how
they live in the world. As they become more energetically
aligned and grounded, their consciousness naturally
expands. These inner changes transform how they
perceive their outer world. Thus, helping people suffer
less emotionally and physically, healing changes
consciousness and is of great service to the world.

This is another reason healing work still makes great
sense to me after all these years. Without so much egoic
drive, the practice is so much simpler, and so much more
powerful.

A client who had been receiving monthly healings for
the last two years told me about a moment when she
became aware of this shift. We were checking in before
her session and she looked straight into my eyes and said
slowly:

"I was playing a friendly game of cards with my

*husband, and I was losing. Then I realized I was
playing the old way. I started playing differently, and
I started to win."*

She didn't have to explain to me what she meant by "differently." She had connected with me on a deeper level before she spoke.

Differently meant playing kinesthetically, instinctively, fully present in the moment, thoroughly engaging both sides of the brain. Differently meant intuitively, not just thinking about what the best card to play next is, but sensing it with her whole being. Differently meant flowhacking. Playing differently requires much less effort. The difference in playing the "old way" and playing "differently" is a very profound, yet subtle shift in awareness.

She said "differently" was much more fun.

25

WE ARE ALL CONNECTED

I HAVE AN INTELLIGENT, VERY CONSCIOUS ANIMAL-LOVING
friend who is a holistic healing practitioner and speaks
three languages. She is the person I ask to edit the posts I
write for my online healing blog. She is especially helpful
when I am trying to write about the more mysterious
nature of energy work, and I am worried I am getting too
far out in left field.

This friend has a very fine-tuned New Age bullshit
meter. If she likes the post, I don't have to worry that I'm
being too woo-woo.

A few years ago she went to a highly respected medi-
tation/coaching conference and came back with an
amazing observation.

The workshop was in a beautiful retreat center
surrounded by trees, with large windows in the main
gathering space. When the thirty participants were meditating in a heart-centered circle, she noticed the strong
winds outside stopped blowing. Everything became calm,
and when the meditation was over, the wind would pick

up again. It happened more than once over the course of the five-day workshop.

She had opened to a new level of energetic awareness and possible human potential.

I have found that every time we gather together and meditate, pray, chant or share a healing session, we are affecting everything around us. The peace, the love, and the healing energy we connect with in the session affects the whole planet. We have no idea of how powerful we are.

I can feel this at my office in my Oakland neighborhood—the birds outside my window, the activity in the streets—reflect the energy of each session. The healing space itself has become a calming vortex of peace.

We are all connected.

26

EVERY HUMAN BEING HAS A UNIQUE WAY OF EXPERIENCING ENERGY

I WILL NEVER FORGET THIS MOMENT.

Early one afternoon I was preparing the healing room for the next session while listening to a radio show called *Seeing Beyond*. There were two guests that day talking to Bonnie Coleen about spiritual house cleaning. One was James Van Praagh, who describes himself as a clairvoyant and spiritual medium and has written many books including *Ghosts Among Us*, *Talking to Heaven*, and *Reaching to Heaven*. The other was Mary Ann Winkowski, a paranormal investigator from Ohio who can talk with ghosts. Mary Ann Winkowski wrote an interesting book about her life, abilities, and paranormal experiences called *When Ghosts Speak*.

In the few minutes it took to get the room in order, they explained how Mary Ann could only see ghosts who were earth bound, and James could only see spirits that had crossed over.

I stood frozen for several minutes after I heard this. This was fascinating. I realized intuition was not just one blanket skill. They were both mediums, which is a specific ability, yet in that distinct skill they each had quite different levels of perception.

I realized healers are like this too. In fact, everyone has their own unique way of perceiving and working with energy and intuitive information. Some people are kinesthetic. (I raise my hand). Some practitioners feel energy emotionally; some people see energy; and some people work with spirit guides, spirits, and angels. Energy shows up perfectly for the specific healer.

This insight also clued me into how differently my clients perceive energy and what meditations and exercises would best support them between sessions. Some clients would be best able to ground themselves by standing barefoot on the earth and others would benefit more from doing a grounding visualization.

Being aware of how my clients experience their life force energy makes it so much easier to help them self-heal and share the practices they would actually do. The best meditations are the ones the client will actually do.

27

PERCEPTION OF SOUND AND
ENERGETIC ALIGNMENT

The nonjudgmental space I had discovered in my healings eventually started to show up in my life. This didn't happen right away, and for many years there seemed to be a lag in what I became aware of in my healing/meditation sessions and the rest of my life outside the healing space. Sometimes this was extremely uncomfortable.

It eventually did integrate especially after the month-long retreat of 2018. My life now does flow much more effortlessly from work to home to everything else. Playing with sound has made this flow much smoother. Sound has become a useful form of self-care, along with Self-Reiki, Breathwork sessions, Healing Touch treatments, and regular exercise.

Guidance often comes to me by a thought that just keeps reoccurring. Learning the difference between an obsessive thought and what may be my higher wisdom still needs time to reveal itself. The desire to explore sound, ocarinas, singing bowls, flutes, and drums has turned out to be a divine gift, even though it first felt like an excessive urge. Excessive and relentless.

I do not actually use tuning forks, singing bowls, flutes, drums or other sound tools in my healing practice with clients. There are already too many things going on in my sessions just using my intention and hands. Yet, playing and exploring sound and these instruments has greatly impacted my healing practice.

One day a client and I were checking in before her session, and I asked if she had noticed any shifts in her life since her last appointment. The first thing she said was, "Yes, music sounded so amazing for three days after that last session."

As I mentioned before, regular Reiki, Healing Touch and Breathwork treatments align and organize our energy fields. When we are centered and grounded, we begin to experience our world differently. Our perception of music, pitch, and acoustics can also become more sensitive when we are in the present moment and in balance. Our inner world changes how we hear our outer world.

There are times when I can hear, sing, and play exactly the right note or chord, and other times I just can't hear it. I don't know how "musically sensitive" I am at any giving moment until I actually try to play an instrument or sing. I still find this to be so strange.

I realized this perceptional shift many years ago in my healing practice. Before every healing session, I always organize the room and set the energy specifically for each client. I feel each session is a private ceremony. I select the sheets, pillows, water glass, and sage/incense that each client prefers. The temperature of the room is important. Some people like a warmer healing space, others like a cooler room. Music is always a large part of this process. The music is carefully selected and playing when the client walks in.

I want to note here that there are times when I just don't know what music to play. I have to wait until my client arrives and feel out what they need. Sometimes I have to change the music I had originally selected after they arrive.

I cannot tell you how many times I have started a healing session, and as soon as I ground into the energy I suddenly become aware that the music is WAY TOO LOUD.

It is always startling. How could I have set the music level at such a high volume? I am so careful. I really pay attention and even set the music a little lower than what I perceive because I am aware that I am more sensitive in the healing space. It still happens every so often, even after over twenty years of setting the volume of the music, that I am way off. I find it so fascinating that I am so much more sensitive to sound when in the healing state. My clients often report the same experience.

Sound for me is a big part of my self-care.

Sound has a great effect on my own energy. Before a workday of healing I often play one of my ocarinas and feel the grounding effect it has on my own body. I often play one long note and feel it resonate internally, as well as hear it. Everyday I resonate to a different note or group of notes, a different flute, or ocarina. It doesn't take long; most of the time I feel a difference in a few minutes. It is amazing how the sound affects my whole being. With the double chamber ocarinas I can play with beat phenomena, sympathetic vibration, harmonics, and overtones. If you are curious, there is a list of my two favorite instrument makers in the back of the book.

At this point in my healing practice I am now feeling/hearing sounds in my body when I meditate. My kinesthetic abilities are still constantly evolving, still connected to the also evolving collective flow. In the beginning of this book I wrote about how I can feel frequencies in my client's body. I believe this ability is a direct result of playing with my sound tools.

Toning, humming, drumming, and chanting has been such a grounding bridge between the many states of consciousness I go through as a healer.

I once read many years ago (I wish I had bookmarked it) how entering the great cathedrals can balance your body's energy field. A church built in alignment with sacred geometry resonates those harmonic frequencies and creates sacred space. If our energy field is missing any specific frequencies, the sacred space will fill us with what we need. The holes in your personal biofield are filled and aligned with the vibrations of the architecture.

A space that is holy enables us to become whole. When we are whole, we can self-heal.

28

WHAT IS HEALING?

Stan came to me many years ago. His first session changed his life. He was sixty years old and had been suffering from debilitating anxiety for about forty years. He was often incapacitated with panic attacks for months at a time.

Stan had been persuaded by a friend to come see me even though he obviously did not think highly of energy work. He had tried many things over the years and at this point was quite angry and frustrated. He didn't think anything would help him.

In fact, Stan was so irritated when he arrived that I moved as quickly though the process of filling out the intake forms as I could and got him on the table.

Stan was intimidating. He did not move one muscle during the session. This was a treatment in which my complete trust in the healing process came in really handy, because Stan had a lot of anger in his energy field. I watched the thoughts "I really hope this healing works" and "If he doesn't feel anything he is going to become unglued" roll through my mind. I observed but did not attach to these thoughts. Because I trusted the energy I knew that what ever happened was going to be perfect and maybe this just wasn't his day to heal.

That session consisted of one long chakra connection. When I was finished he lay unmoving on the table for a few minutes while I sat back on my stool. He was so unresponsive I started thinking it might be best not to charge him and get him out of my office as soon as possible. Then he opened his eyes and said, "I have never been so relaxed."

That was unexpected. His anxiety attacks stopped after that session for three months. After a few more sessions they stopped for a longer time.

Then one day something triggered another round of anxiety. Stan called me thinking that something was wrong. I asked how long the anxiety had lasted. He said three days on and off. I reminded him that three days is better than three months, what he had experienced before he first came for a healing. I reminded him that healing was progress.

I explained healing is often not about never having another anxiety attack, stomach ache, or migraine ever again. Healing is not about staying in perfect energetic alignment all the time. It is about being able to reground and recenter as quickly as possible when symptoms arise, as soon as we are triggered.

We are humans living in very interesting times. There is always something that will throw us out of alignment. Like the news, a death in the family, or finding out you owe a lot of taxes. Healing is about how quickly we can find our center again.

29

BARBARA'S HEALING THEORY: ENERGY THERAPY CHANGES THE ENERGETIC PATTERN

I FOUND AN ARTICLE ON THE PERSONAL WEBSITE OF Healing Touch Practitioner Barbara Litchfield, HTCP, MA, CCA, QTP many years ago. I share the excerpt below, with permission. It is a brilliant perspective on the healing process.

Several people have asked this question: "Why don't the effects of the energy work last longer?"

By "effects," they mean relaxation, release of pain, feelings of peacefulness and calm, reduced insomnia among many others.

By "last longer" they may mean a period of time longer than a few days.

The best way to answer this question is by an example.

Suppose I take a thick rubber band and hold it taut between my thumb and index finger. And let's say for the sake of this example that I can do my work and daily activities holding the rubber band as described. It's a bit uncomfortable but not so much that I have to take it off. Well, over time holding the rubber band like this gradually feels awkward, interferes with my activities, and may even cause me some pain.

Being a proponent of holistic health, I seek the services of an energy therapist. She completes the interview, does the assessment of the energy field and chakras, and provides the energetic techniques that address my discomfort. At the end of the session, I'm feeling relaxed, calm, and my pain has decreased.

What I have forgotten is that I had been holding that rubber band between my fingers for over a month while doing what I normally do. . . work at a job, swim, walk my dog, golf, and bike.

My energy field and physical body have developed a pattern to accommodate the holding of this rubber band. What the energy practitioner is beginning to do is *change the energetic pattern.*

Like a chiropractor, the Healing Touch practitioner will ask the client to return in a week to determine if the new energetic pattern has "held." More times than not, it takes several sessions of energy work to clear and balance the field by changing the pattern.

30

CLARITY BREATHWORK

I LOOK BACK ON MY LIFE AT THIS POINT AND SEE IT IN TWO chapters: before Clarity Breathwork and after Clarity Breathwork.

Breathwork was how I cured myself of migraines.

Clarity Breathwork is the practice of circular, connected breathing for healing and attaining higher states of consciousness.

In a breathwork session, the client is comfortably lying on a massage table, fully clothed, and breathes deeply for a full hour. As oxygen fills the body and raises the client's vibration, anything of a lower vibration becomes conscious and can then be released. This includes emotions, past trauma, unconscious beliefs, and habitual physical patterns. Clarity Breathwork connects us with a higher aspect of ourselves so we can let go of shame and blame, and move into self-acceptance, compassion, and love.

I found Clarity Breathworker Maggie Ostara from a postcard advertising her practice. In 2006 she charged

$150.00 for a private session. Back then that seemed outrageously expensive. I thought I could not afford that, so my first Breathwork experience was in her Breathing Circle. In that first breathe I knew that Breathwork was a direct route to releasing my migraines.

I was shocked at what happened in that first breathe. The whole right side of my body tightened up and went into spasms throughout most of the breathe, while the left side of my body felt almost normal. It was so physically intense, it was insane. Yet, I was thrilled because I knew this pattern was connected to my headaches. The right side of my body always contracted the day before the onset of a migraine.

After that first circle, I signed up for private sessions with Maggie Ostara, ready do whatever it took to pay for it. I ended up breathing with her every two weeks for seventeen private breath session and attended every Breath Circle she held. Those sessions changed me and my experience of life. The intensity of my migraines greatly decreased during the first five sessions, and with additional changes in diet and exercise, I was headache free in about a year.

In addition to working with Maggie, I also started breathing with Ashanna Solaris's CD, *Healing Yourself with Breath* everyday for months. I. Love. This. CD. I was committed. Pain is so motivating.

I still breathe with this *Healing Yourself with Breath* CD whenever I feel triggered, emotional, or frustrated. I have listened to this CD more that any other guided meditation or piece of music in my library. I still hear words and affirmations from Ashanna during my breathes that I swear I had never heard her say before.

It's an oracle breathe—I get guidance for that specific day.

I also breathe when my shoulders and back feel tight or tired. Breathing has kept my physical body relaxed, clear, and energized. Breathwork keeps my body strong and flexible; it extended my massage practice at least five years.

I use Clarity Breathwork as a meditation, prayer, and as a major part of my daily meditative practices. Sometimes I do a more traditional meditation before or after breathing, and sometimes I breath with yoga or other energetic practices. I pay for private Breathwork sessions at least every three weeks. Breathwork is flat out amazing.

This is an interesting note: The space I hold in a Breathwork session is different that the space I experience in the energy healing sessions. In this book I have focused on the energetic healing space of my Reiki and Healing Touch clients, not on how I hold the space for my Breathwork clients.

Once in a workshop I was paired with a woman who was trying to release some childhood trauma and she couldn't connect with her trauma when I was holding a healing space for her. I was really surprised to learn that my energy could override her trauma.

One of the benefits of Breathwork is that it brings up the trauma in our physical body to be released. I have learned how to hold a safe and supportive energetic container for my clients in Breathwork sessions. A space where they can also access their trauma to heal and release it. It's a subtle yet very important difference in being a facilitator of the two modalities—breathwork versus energetic healing.

In the Breathwork sessions my clients often have so much physical release I also have to be ready at any moment to keep them from literally falling off the table.

I also use touch as a way of keeping them connected with their bodies when that appears to be helpful. Every session is different, but in general this is what happens.

For me, Breathwork is a spiritual process that connects me to that infinite source of all that is in this moment, in each breath. It was my main go-to therapy for those "dark night of the soul" years.

I can tangibly feel it—that experience of being connected to all that is and that space makes everything okay. My heart expands and there is so much joy. This is the one healing space I feel emotion. The more I access this feeling, this dimension, the easier it is for me to be present in my body and in my life. This incredibly real and physical experience of the universal life energies is the greatest healer of all.

31

CHECKING IN: SHOULD I WORK TODAY?

DOING ENERGY WORK FIVE DAYS A WEEK MEANS THAT eventually you will wake up and have an off day. It could be an emotional, mental, or physical issue.

In the first ten years of my practice, I had low-grade migraines so frequently that it would have been impossible for me to keep my business going if I didn't work on the off days that were due to the migraines. So I had to check in many mornings.

To check in, I usually I sit down, ground, and ask myself slowly, "Should I work today?" I form the words in my head one at a time. Then I wait for my body, my being, and inner knowing to respond.

If I feel calm, that is a yes. If I feel stressed, that is a no. It sounds so simple, but this simple process has helped me immensely. I hope it might help you.

When I do have an off day, for whatever reason, I immediately start looking at my schedule and start blocking off time in the immediate future to recharge.

If I feel I might be contagious, or like I am coming down with something, I do call and cancel with my client immediately.

32

MASSAGE

I LOVE MASSAGE. I LOVE GIVING MASSAGE AND I LOVE receiving massage. I learned so much about healing and consciousness as a Massage Therapist. Being a Massage Therapist is an amazing, beautiful journey. I really miss my massage sessions and clients.

Massage taught me how to start and sustain a healing business. As a massage therapist, I learned so much about taking money, scheduling, setting up my healing office, how to take care of myself, and how to file my taxes. I released a lot of fear around asking for money and how money is just another form of energy.

Being a Massage Therapist was one of the greatest things that ever happened to me. Eventually though, it can become physically challenging and you have to let it go. For my healer/clients who want to transition from massage therapist to healer I first remind them how sacred the massage space is.

I recommend that they acknowledge every massage as a powerful healing, the most powerful healing possible in that moment. Express gratitude for the session and all the possibilities available in that moment. Hold everything that arises with great compassion, even your own resistance.

I found this to be the most direct path to creating the healing practice you want.

33

TRAINING, CERTIFICATIONS, AND WORKSHOPS

HOW MANY MODALITIES, CERTIFICATIONS, AND TRAININGS do you need to do healing work? The real answer is none. Healing is an inherent ability we all have.

If you are starting a healing practice now with the intention of financially supporting yourself, I recommend beginning with one certification in an established modality. A solid program like Healing Touch, Healing Beyond Borders, or Reiki with fantastic teachers such as Frans Stiene and Kathleen Prasad. Check out the local teachers your local area. There are so many great teachers and programs out there. See the Resource section for a list.

Because I wanted to be a "professional" I needed to know everything; it was part of that spiritual seeking drive I had. I started with Healing Touch, a program that was as intense as graduate school.

I am "certified" in three modalities: Clarity Breathwork, Healing Touch, and Reiki. I think of my practice as having two modalities: Breathwork and energetic healing.

I also was trained in massage. That means I have taken all the classes, done all the coursework, have my certificates of completion, and stay current with the teachings. This is total overkill.

On a business and marketing level, I find it advantageous to have a solid foundation in two different modalities. Each modality has a community and the crossover referrals are extremely helpful. My Breathwork community has friends healing from cancer and they know that supporting people through cancer is one of the focuses of my healing practice. Many people in my Healing Touch community have also tried Breathwork.

There are some excellent energetic practitioners out there who have been certified with every modality under the sun—and that is great. For me, even though I studied every modality I could find, I found the fees, website upkeep, and recertifications too much to keep up with. The Clarity Breathwork, Reiki, and Healing Touch community provides me with all the support I need in this moment.

That being said, I am studying Eileen Day McKusick's visionary work with tuning forks and vibration, reading her blogs, articles, and watching her YouTube videos. I am still a workshop junkie, but it is much more fun now.

I really needed the solid foundation of Healing Touch when I started my practice. Without this solid foundation I would have never had the confidence to, as Healing Touch founder Janet Mentgen said, "Just do the Work."

Healing Touch is how "Doing The Work" evolved into "Being The Work."

34

HEALING IN HOSPITALS

MANY OF THE "MIRACLE SESSIONS" I HAVE EXPERIENCED with my clients have been in hospitals. Getting energetic healing modalities such as Reiki and Healing Touch into our medical institutions would eliminate so much suffering and promote vital self-healing. If there is one way this book may influence the world may it be to encourage energetic healing in hospitals. Even one healing session in a hospital can create enough energetic support to turn a patient's healing process around. Energy healing in hospitals would greatly shift our medical culture.

My first guideline in going into hospitals as an energy practitioner is that you work around the medical staff and their schedule. You are there to support them, and they are part of the healing.

When a nurse arrives to take blood from my client in the middle of my healing, I always look her in the eye and energetically invite her into the room as soon as I notice her or him. I am holding the healing space for her and every hospital worker who comes into the room. Often the nurses volunteer to come back later when they realize there is a healing happening. I have been in many hospitals over the years, hired by the patients, and the nurses have always been very supportive of the healing work.

I have found that holding a healing space for the patient is the easiest part of holding space in a hospital. It's the family that can throw you off. Emotions can run high when a family member is sick. I have to be careful to stay grounded with the high frequencies of the healing and fearful family members. I find my focus is sometimes on the family members as much as the patient. This is where I focus on holding everything in the moment with great compassion. We are talking rubber meeting the road here.

In a hospital room, attitudes can be so thick you can cut them with a knife. People can think you are a New Age nut, taking hard earned money from their family, or taking advantage of their loved one's illness. For me, those are the easier attitudes to navigate than the family members who think I am going to "save" their mom, or son, or other loved one—that is most difficult for me. Some people consider healers miracle workers.

I find it so much easier to deal with skeptics.

If someone is paying me to come to the hospital I usually do a full hands-on-healing. At this point I don't need to put my hands on someone to create a space for miracles to arrive, but it's an easy way to figure out which "form" the healing needs to take to connect with the patient.

People are usually watching you do the session in a hospital too, so it is easier to look like something is happening. Some clients just need touch, especially in a hospital bed. Some people feel really connected to more prayer-like healings. The energy lets me know what is required.

I also want to say that *everyone* can hold space in the hospital for themselves or a loved one. Prayer, meditation, or pujas are all so helpful. Even when it does not feel like you are doing anything, let me assure you that you are. You will feel it, experience it, and know it on a deep level the more you do it.

One grounded centered person can shift the energy of an entire room.

We. Are. More. Powerful. Than. We. Have. Ever. Imagined.

35

CHEMOTHERAPY AND RADIATION

ONCE I WAS CERTIFIED IN HEALING TOUCH, I FOUND energy work to be incredibly effective in supporting people through radiation and chemotherapy. I have had so many people walk into my office suffering from the side effects of chemotherapy and have had them walk out feeling so much better physically and emotionally. This includes pain, nausea, fatigue, anxiety, and neuropathy. As I saw Healing Touch make such a big difference in the quality of life of these clients, I chose to make supporting these clients the focus of my healing practice for many years.

I had the idea when I started working with people diagnosed with cancer that before and after each chemotherapy infusion would be the best time for them to get a healing. I was taught the more healings the better.

This was just not practical. I now charge $150.00 per healing and not all clients can afford that. I also discovered that clients with a cancer diagnosis are very busy people. Many are taking care of families and many are still working, as well as adding hospital visits and doctor appointments to their schedules. People receiving chemotherapy are also tired. The fewer appointments they have, the more rest they can get.

Healing sessions right after chemotherapy appeared to be the most potent time for my clients. That was when clearing and assisting them in energetically organizing their biofield benefited them the most. The more organized their energy field, the less chemo is needed. The less chemo, the less side effects.

I learned so much, through observation and a clear intention to help others. I still had a lot of egoic I'm-going-to-make-you-better desire to make a difference in my client's lives. Yet, I was still open to seeing what worked and what did not work.

I wrote about what I discovered in an article in "Supporting Clients Going Through Chemotherapy," *Energy Magazine*, Nov/Dec 2016, Issue Eighty-Eight. If you are energetically supporting someone healing from cancer this is a good article to read. Then follow your own direct experience.

36

THE BUSINESS OF HEALING

THERE ARE A LOT OF COACHES, COURSES AND BUSINESS groups out there that want to help you develop your business practice for a large initial investment. I suggest you take your time when committing to these programs and consider all your options.

The marketing strategy that was the most effective in my business was word-of-mouth. Starting and sustaining a healing practice is a very organic process that changes you from the inside out. What you think you want now will probably not be what you want in a year. Trust your intuition and watch how every step unfolds.

I have worked with many people who wanted to be healers and who realized a year or so into the process that having a healing business was not for them. Yet, the process of doing energy work opened them to new possibilities in their lives they would never have found without practicing energy work.

Whatever you decide to do in your life, studying and working with energy will benefit you in ways you may never have imagined. Daily self-treatments alone make a huge difference in your life.

How your practice best integrates into your life unfolds as you do the work. Do you like working in the morning? Only three days a week? Do you like maintaining an office? How much money do you need/want to make? Do you want to do outcalls? Do you like working with clients diagnosed with cancer? Or children, or animals? How many clients can you see in a day? How much time do you schedule between sessions?

Being self-employed is not for everyone. There are many ways to be a professional healer in this world. You can work in a retreat center, yoga studio, clinic, or hospital.

One woman I worked with who was a wonderful healer and already certified in Healing Touch wanted to leave her full-time job as a nurse. I gave her a list of things to do: get a business card, get a one-page website—all simple business things. As she completed each round of assignments, we met again and discussed how her practice was growing. I then gave her another list. She had all the work she wanted in a fairly short time. Then I stopped hearing from her.

Some time later, I called her to check in and she told me she decided not to have a healing business at this time in her life. She had incorporated her Healing Touch into her job and she was now excited about doing the work in the hospital where she worked. That was many years ago and since then she has brought so much comfort to so many people and is fully engaged in her job.

One aspect of having a healing practice that has been

the most paradoxical for me is marketing. Healing is a mystery. Marketing a mystery is tricky. How do I explain to people how beneficial energy healing is when I can't guarantee an outcome? When I have let go of expectations, outcomes, and results?

I started a blog as an attempt to verbalize the things that happened in my sessions in ways people might understand. Some posts took me *months* to write because I had to process on some nonverbal level what is essentially indescribable. Believe it or not, I found explaining the unexplainable got easier. I hope my blog has made it easier for other practitioners to write about their practice.

Commitment to life means taking action to materialize your dreams. Dreams change and evolve as they manifest. Everything unfolds in perfect timing.

37

THE GIFT OF AWE

I AM IN AWE OF ALL MY CLIENTS. WHEN I AM FULLY PRESENT with someone, from when I first meet them at my office door and sit at the table before they get on the healing table, I can feel their light, their true self—whatever you want to call it.

My clients are so intelligent, successful, courageous, and magnificent, it inspires me. They feel my awareness of their true essence and begin to feel it in themselves. I believe that seeing this light, this inner beauty and all its manifestations, is one of my gifts as a healer.

The ability to see my client's true self and hold a grounded space for them to heal is because I can completely trust and follow the energy.

All healers are different. I hope that by writing about my process of learning about my healing abilities, I can support you in finding your own unique gifts.

EPILOGUE

*There is a great freedom and relief when the search for
what we imagine is lacking comes to an end (not
forever after, but right now.) What remains is the
simplicity of being just this moment, exactly as it is—
just this! Ever-changing, unresolvable, ungraspable,
unavoidable. Instead of trying to formulate or
transcend it, this is an invitation to simply BE it.*

- Joan Tollifson

May this book bring you valuable insights into your own
healing practice, consciousness, and life.

ACKNOWLEDGMENTS

I would like to thank Beth Barany, my writing coach who met with me for over a year while I wrote this book. Beth is a genius. Without Beth, these words would have never made it to the page.

I want to thank my mom, Barbara Lawson, for all her support, especially for holding such a high space when we were sheltering in. I would like to thank my awe-inspiring sister Janet and my nephew Jasper, one of the most beautiful humans on the planet.

Carol Kinney, my Healing Touch Mentor all those years ago.

Thank you Marci Laughlin, Teri Duff, and Yolanda Calderon, for your valuable feed back on the manuscript.

Thank you Barbara Litchfield for allowing me to share your article on changing energetic patterns.

Sophia Arise, thank you for all your insightful suggestions in writing the book and all the Breathwork sessions you have given me. I am so grateful for your friendship and support.

Thank you, Heather Swallow, for trusting your gifts and being such a light in with world. You are a superhero.

Thank you Nicki Boisvert for your insights, writings and depth of being.

Thank you to Terese Allara and Neal Lowen. You have provided me and so many others the space to do art and healing work in Oakland, California. Your building is a vortex of great creative and healing energy. Your support, friendship and love has been a great support over the years.

Thank you Healing Touch community. May we continue to share our light.

I want to thank all my clients. Every session has been a gift.

Thank you Geoffrey Matsumoto for your presence, wisdom, and love.

RESOURCES

BOOKS AND ARTICLES

Reiki

Reiki For Dogs by Kathleen Prasad, Ulysses Press: Berkeley, California 2012

The Inner Heart of Reiki Rediscovering Your True Self by Frans Stiene, Ayni Books 2015

Healing

"Supporting Clients Going Through Chemotherapy" by Jeri Lawson, *Energy Magazine*, Nov/Dec 2016, Issue Eighty-Eight

When Ghosts Speak: Understanding the World of Earthbound Spirits by Mary Ann Winkowski, Grand Central Publishing, 2009

Sound

Tuning the Human Biofield Healing with Vibrational Sound Therapy by Eileen Day McKusick, Healing Arts Press: Rochester, Vermont 2014

If you are interested in sound healing, this book is a very good place to start.

Songbird Ocarinas

Check out the Seedpod Bass In C and The Seedpod Ocarina G
https://www.songbirdocarina.com/

Stonewhistle

https://stonewhistle.com/
Han's website is fascinating.

Non-duality and Spirituality

A New Earth: Awakening To Your Life's Purpose by Eckart Tolle, Walker and Company: New York NY 2008

Death: The End Of Self Improvement by Joan Tollif-

son, New Sarum Press Salisbury, United Kingdom
2019

Whatever Arises, Love That: A Love Revolution That Begins with You by Matt Kahn, Sounds True 2016

Essence Revisited: Slipping Past the Shadows of Illusion by Darryl Bailey, Darryl Bailey & Non-Duality Press May 2011

One of my favorite Non-duality writers. I recommend everything he has written.

The Way Of Liberation: A Practical Guide To Spiritual Enlightenment By Adyashanti, Open Gate Sangha San Jose, California 2012

ORGANIZATIONS, WEBSITES, AND HEALING PROGRAMS

Animal Reiki Source

https://www.animalreikisource.com/

Kathleen Prasad's teaching website with links to Animal Reiki classes, articles, blog, meditations and world directory of Animal Reiki Practitioners. I highly recommend taking at least one class with Kathleen and learn the form of Reiki she now calls Let Animals Lead®. Kathleen is a skilled teacher and a Master Reiki Practitioner. Just being around her for a few days will open you energetically to your own inherent healing potentials. This is ground breaking consciousness work and a good core foundation.

Kathleen's Shelter Animal Reiki Association (SARA)

https://shelteranimalreikiassociation.org/

An incredible non-profit organization founded by Kathleen Prasad and Leah D'Ambrosio that teaches and promotes the Let Animals Lead® method of Reiki to shelter and sanctuary animals. SARA works closely with staff and volunteers using meditation and healing practices to help create a positive healing space for all. SARA volunteers don't do Reiki to Animals, they are Reiki with the Animals.

The International House Of Reiki

https://ihreiki.com

The website of Frans Stiene and Bronwen Logan (Stiene). Frans has studied and teaches the traditional Japanese approach to Reiki as a path of spiritual development and healing. A great core energetic foundation for all healers, both beginning and advanced. Frans is one of the great Reiki teachers of our time.

Pamela Miles

https://reikiinmedicine.org/

Pamela Miles lives in New York and has written a Reiki blog sine 2009. She is a great promoter of Reiki for self-care and an experienced teacher.

Elizabeth A Fulmer, RMT, SD

Reiki Master/Teacher, Spiritual Director
http://reikifocus.org/

A wonderful human being and gifted Reiki teacher who has ignited a whole community of healers in Davis, California.

Healing Touch

There are two organizations that teach Healing Touch and both are excellent. I am certified by Healing Touch Program.

Healing Touch Program:
https://discover.healingtouchprogram.com/

Healing Beyond Borders:
https://www.healingbeyondborders.org/

Clarity Breathwork

https://claritybreathwork.com/

The websites of my teachers Ashanna Solaris and

Dana Delong. This is the form of Breathwork I facilitate and practice.

Janna Moll, Sem, Msn, Lmt, Htp

Energy Medicine from Energy Medicine Specialists
https://www.energymedicinespecialists.com/

Bengston Energy Healing Method®

"A non-invasive, information-based healing method — developed and rigorously researched by William Bengston, PhD"—From his website.

https://bengstonresearch.com/

I highly recommend all of William Bengston's work. If you can't see him speak in person, definitely check out his book and research. Even though I don't use his cycling technique in my healing work, his research and ideas are right on the edge of what is possible. I personally would love to take another workshop with him.

Supriya Ishaya, Teacher of The Ishaya's Ascension

artofawareness.me

GLOSSARY

BIOFIELD

The biofield is the field of energy/information that surrounds and interpenetrates the human body. Also referred to as "the human energy field" or "aura."

FLOW HACKING

Flow is the optimal state of consciousness where you feel and perform at your best state. There is rapt attention and total focus in the moment, and everything else disappears. Action and awareness merge. You have no sense of individual self. Time slows down or speeds up. Flow hacking is how you get to the flow state, whether it is through surfing, parachuting, skateboarding, ritual, meditation, or healing.

HOLDING SPACE

Holding space means to be with someone without judgment, expectations, or agenda. To listen without interrupting to what another person needs to say or not say.

Energetically in my healing practice I "hold space" for whatever needs to happen for my client. This may mean perfect stillness, waves of emotions, physical releases, spirit guide intervention, and altered states of consciousness.

NONDUALITY

The nature of reality in which there are not two, but the experience of one. No subject-object. The experience or knowing of a reality that is unified and much more vast than the reality of our daily lives. The realization that form and reality are not separate, as waves are not separate from the ocean. The understanding that all things are interconnected.

OCARINA

The ocarina is an ancient wind musical instrument traditionally made from clay or ceramic. Ocarinas can have four to twelve finger holes and a mouthpiece that projects from the enclosed body of the instrument. There are many creative variations of ocarinas made from plastic, glass, wood, metal, or bone. They are also made with many different tunings, shapes, and number of sound holes.

PUJA

Pūjā" is a Sanskrit word meaning worship, honor, and reverence. A Puja is a ritual usually consisting of a loving offering of light, flowers, food, and water to the divine. Puja is an essential ritual of Hinduism.

UNITY CONSCIOUSNESS

The state of consciousness where everything is connected.

ABOUT THE AUTHOR

Jeri Lawson is a Clarity Breathwork, Reiki, and Healing Touch Practitioner with a full-time practice in Oakland, California for over twenty-five years. She is a graduate of Psychic Horizons Clairvoyant Program, the National Holistic Institute, and has also studied Shamanism, Depth Hypnosis, Craniosacral Therapy, and Matrix Energetic and the Bengston Energy Healing Method®.

Her intention as a healer is to assist her clients in bringing their energy field into balance so they can heal themselves. She knows energetic healing and breathwork can connect us to our deepest inner guidance and inherent healing ability.

In her book she states:

> *"My intention is not to tell you how to heal, or what you should experience in a session, but to give you the confidence to let the energy guide you in opening to your unique abilities as you start your healing practice. What you think should happen and what actually happens in a healing could be very different things. The direct experience of your healing sessions is where you can discover the portal to that healing place where all possibilities exist—the possibilities for you and your client."*

To find out more about Jeri Lawson's practice, check out her site: https://jerilawsonhealingtouch.com/.